Run Your
Bad Habits Away

Beginner Running Guide
From 0-5k And Beyond

Table of Contents

Introduction

Running is one of the best ways to get fit, strong and healthy. For one, it's probably the most practical form of meaningful regular exercise because all you need are a good pair of running shoes and socks, a good pair of running shorts, a good quality running shirt and road! You can also do it practically anytime and anywhere, as roads are open 24/7! You also don't have to wait until other people are ready and available to do your regular runs because running is an individual sport. In fact, running with your buddies may even be an unwanted distraction, unless you and your friends are disciplined enough to focus on the running part more than on the social interaction part. And the best part of it all, at least for me, is the increased levels of happy hormones called endorphins. Running regularly helps you have more of them and, as a result, you feel much happier most of the time. It's like being on happy drugs - the natural, safe and legal way!

In other words, you won't have any excuse not to get fit and healthy through regular running other than laziness.

In this book, you will learn about the most important basic principles of running first. Simply following a running training plan - no matter how good it is - won't cut it because without a good understanding of the underlying principles, you may not be able to execute the training plan optimally or worse, you may even get injured or sick, which are the complete opposites of what you're trying to accomplish through running. Only after the basic principles have been explained will I elaborate on a 12-week running plan that will have you - a total newbie - up and running your first 5 kilometer run. And if you continue building up on the progress that you made using the principles I'll share here, you'll be able to run longer both in terms of time and distance. In the process, you'll become fitter, stronger and healthier.

So, let's cut to the chase and get on with the principles already.

Chapter 1 - The Habit Factor

Power of habit

"Motivation is what gets you started. Habit is what keeps you going." – Jim Ryan

The fact that you bought this book and are reading it already means that you have the motivation to start running in order to get fit, strong and healthy. But it wouldn't be wise to rely on motivation to keep you going long enough to make running a normal part of your lifestyle and to become and ultimately stay fit, strong and healthy. You'll need something else to help keep you running for the long term. And that something is habit.

Loosely defined, habit is an action that has become normal for you. This means you don't have to think about or remember to do something regularly just so you do it frequently enough. To use a simpler term, a habit is an action that is automatic or runs on autopilot.

Habit is better than motivation because when the physical conditions surrounding your running become bad or very challenging, you don't need to use up much of your willpower just to get through it. If running becomes a habit for you, it will actually be more challenging for you and more taxing on your will power to not run on certain days. Think of it this way - smoking is a very bad health habit that millions of people have. And because it has become an ingrained habit for these people, they find it very, very hard, if not impossible, to stop the habit even if they know that it's very bad for their health. So, can you imagine if something as healthy as running becomes a strongly ingrained habit for you? Go figure.

But this is not to say that motivation is totally useless. May it never be my friend! What I'm trying to say here is that motivation should not be your foundation but should only serve as a catalyst at the start and support system over the long term when it comes to running for health, fitness and physical strength.

The Art of Developing Habits

When it comes to developing or ingraining a habit, there are a couple of things that can prove to be very helpful to you: Planning, consistency, motivation and accountability. Let's talk about planning first.

It has been said that failing to plan is planning to fail. I totally agree with that saying. The main reason why there's much truth to this saying is risk, which can be defined as the chance or probability that something undesirable will happen. When you don't plan well or when you don't plan at all, your risk of not being able to achieve the things you want to do become substantially higher. Conversely, planning well lowers such risks and increases your chances of successfully achieving your goals, which in this case is to make running properly a habit.

So how does proper planning allow you to do that? Proper planning allows you to anticipate much, if not all, possible challenges and obstacles that may arise as you pursue your goals. For example, one of the most challenging aspects of training to run longer is making time for it. You can either run first thing in the morning before going to work or school, or you can run later in the afternoon or early evening as soon as your work is done. But for you to increase your chances of being able to have available time either in the morning or in the evening, you will need to anticipate possible problems or challenges that can deprive you of such running times.

For example, if you choose to run first thing in the morning, you will need to consider the fact that you will need to run very early so you can have enough time to freshen up, eat a healthy breakfast, and get to work or school on time. To maximize your chances of being able to wake up early and have enough energy to run in the morning, you will need to hit the sack earlier at night. So, part of proper planning for this is making sure that on most evenings, you can go to bed early. And if there are possible obstacles to this, planning properly will not just help you identify these possible obstacles but also to find ways to either eliminate them or get around them so you can sleep earlier.

The second important thing that can help you successfully develop the habit running properly is consistency. Another way to define the word habit is what Mahatma Gandhi once said: *"Your beliefs become your thoughts. Your thoughts become your words. Your words become your actions. Your actions become your habits. Your habits become your values. Your values become your destiny."* And I would like to emphasize the middle portion which says what you normally do eventually becomes your habit. In other words, action that is done repetitively becomes a habit. When you plan accordingly, your chances of repeating a certain action frequently enough is optimized.

So how frequently should you repeat a specific action or practice in order to make it become a habit? The truth is it really depends on the nature of the habit to be acquired and the person acquiring the habit. But on average, it takes about 21 straight days of performing a desired habit for it to start gaining traction and become more and more automatic. And on this first 21 days, you'll need to muster all the motivation and willpower that you can get to ensure consistency.

And speaking of motivation, this is the third component of developing a habit. Remember the quote from Jim Ryan at the start of the chapter? There are many different ways to motivate yourself and to stay motivated, but none is as effective or powerful than having a very powerful reason for acquiring habit. In his best-selling book "The Power of Habit," Charles Duhigg cited the example of navy seal trainees who were able to successfully finish the navy seals training program, which is one of the hardest if not the hardest training program in the world. It's so hard that only a small portion of the trainees that are accepted into the program ever make it past the finish line. Duhigg noted a particular mental and motivational strategy employed by both the trainers and the trainees that allow them to push beyond their perceived limits and accomplish seemingly superhuman tasks. And what was this strategy or tactic?

They ask themselves why they're doing something as crazy as navy seals training.

Duhigg noted in his book that it is usually the people with the flimsiest or shallowest reasons who drop out from the program. It's because flimsy or shallow reasons are the weakest of motivations. But those whose reasons were deeply personal and significant were able to find enough motivation to power them through the training program. And by the end of that program, doing seemingly superhuman or out of this world tasks that most people would never dare to even try and do has become a habit.

So, if, at some point during the early phases of your running training program, you find things to be very challenging or difficult, remember your significant and deeply personal reasons for training, which is to enjoy a long, fit, strong and healthy life. You can be even more motivated by looking at pictures or watching videos of people suffering from serious chronic or degenerative health conditions as a result of not living a healthy, fit and strong lifestyle. I know it may sound insensitive but the truth is, pain or the fear of massive pain can be amplified by looking at graphic examples what it truly means to suffer from such massive pain.

Accountability is the final piece for helping you optimize your chances of successfully making running and all running related practices a habit. Accountability means being answerable to another person for not being able to do something you committed yourself to do.   Under accountability, you are giving permission or authority to another person to call you out or even impose certain punishments or penalties for not being able to accomplish something you committed to do. You should choose an accountability partner who you know won't shy away from making your life hard every time you fail to do something that you are supposed to do. So, don't go for your friends or family members who are all positive, hopeful or worse, nice. If you really want to succeed in making running and all its related practices a habit, you should choose a drill sergeant-like person for your accountability partner.

Chapter 2 - The Holy Trinity of Training for Results

Consider the tallest building or skyscraper in your city. Have you ever seen it while it was still being constructed? If you happened to pass by the site on a regular basis, you probably have. And when you think about it, you would have noticed that for the longest time, no significant progress was being accomplished during the 1st half or 3/4 of the total construction time and that only during the last half or 1/4 of the construction time where much of the building was finished.

If you thought of it that way, I wouldn't blame you. Most high-rise buildings, especially in major cities or business districts, are constructed with tall makeshift walls surrounding the whole sites, which prevents passersby from actually seeing the work that's being done on the site. What most passers-by don't see, you and I, are the tedious and voluminous amounts of work that were done to establish those buildings' foundations, on which the entire visible building would stand. It can't be done any other way because 80% of a building's ability to stay erect even in the face of earthquakes is dependent on the foundation. The higher the building, the deeper the foundation.

And so, it is when it comes to running - your ability to establish a deep and strong foundation will determine whether or not you can successfully run for the long haul. Running may be akin to a very sharp stainless-steel kitchen knife in that if handled very well, it can yield the most beautiful results and if handled improperly or poorly, it can hurt people badly. By establishing a good knowledge and foundation for running, you'll be able to establish a good practical foundation for it, which will allow you to enjoy running and all its benefits even in old age.

Before The Trinity, a Testament

One of the best books on running is the bestselling classic "Born to Run" by Christopher McDougall. In that book, it was mentioned that running is the only sport where the decline from the peak is at its slowest. Compared to other professional sports where most people retire at the very old age of 30 to 35 years, many people still continue to run marathons even way past their senior age of 60 years old!

Why is that? It's because running using proper form, which we'll tackle later on in detail, makes running the least, if not one of the least, physically stressful sports on the human body. If you look at the NBA in the United States, quite a handful of stars - young ones at that - have already fallen prey to injuries during the first 1/3 of the 2017-2018 regular season. Why? It's because of the immense physical stress that today's level of competition puts on the bodies of NBA players. Vince Carter is already considered a dinosaur at 40 years old, and though while he still has some hop in his legs and moments of brilliance in playing the game at the highest level of basketball competition the world over, he was already very far from his peak when he was in his 20s.

But consider Harriette Thompson, who passed away in October 2017, the oldest woman in history to ever finish a half and a full marathon. In 2015, she officially became the oldest woman to finish a full marathon when she finished the San Diego Rock n' Roll marathon in under 7 1/2 hours - at the age of 92 years and 93 days old! You read that right - 92 years and 93 days old! But wait, there's more!

In June 2017, she became the oldest woman in history to finish a half-marathon when she clocked in at a shade under 3 hours and 43 minutes at age 94. Yes, 94 years old! If a nonagenarian who has survived cancer and only started training for a marathon at age 76 can finish a full marathon, doesn't that tell you that contrary to what many people think, running is a safe sport? I think it does! And the fact that she died because of complications from injuries due to a bad fall and not because of sickness or disease is a testament to how running can help people become much healthier, even after being stricken with cancer!

Now that I've (hopefully) convinced you that running isn't a dangerous sport and that it's something that just about anybody with enough desire, discipline and determination can do, let's tackle the foundational principles of running, a.k.a., the Holy Trinity of running: Training, rest and nutrition.

Chapter 3 - Training

"The hardest step for a runner is the first one out the door." –
Unknown

Why do I even need to learn about how to run? Duh? Even a toddler can do that without having to read a book, watch a YouTube instructional video, or hire a trainer!

I've heard that line before and it's highly possible that, at some point prior to grabbing your copy of this book, you have asked the same question or something like it. Truth is you really don't need to read a book such as this, watch instructional videos, or to hire a trainer in order to run. It's like asking if you need to attend a class on how to breathe. It's a natural and instinctive process!

But there's a big difference between simply being able to run and running optimally. It's easy to run 100 meters on pure instinct for 1 or 2 times but it's a totally different thing to run at least 5 kilometers, finish an official run, finish it strong and get fit in the process. And it's another entirely different thing to do it until you're old and gray - and possibly toothless! You see, running for longevity and fitness requires that you know how to run optimally, which is neither as natural nor as common sense as many people think it is.

And that's why we have this chapter on training properly.

Proper Form

You may not be aware of it but proper form can spell the difference between being able to run until you're old, gray and toothless, and retire from running due to a blown out knee or broken ankle. The most successful runners - like Harriette Thompson - are able to run until their sunset years and enjoy the major health benefits of running because they've managed to minimize the risks or even avoid running related injuries and medical conditions altogether by using proper form. And when talking about form, you'll need to first know what kind of a "striker" are you.

The foot strike refers to how your feet land on the ground as you run. There are 3 general ways people's feet hit the ground during running: heel, mid-foot and forefoot. If you're a heel striker, it means your heels come into contact with the ground first - absorbing the impact of your bodyweight hitting the ground - with each and every stride. If you're a mid-foot and forefoot striker, then the middle of your feet and your forefoot (the balls of your feet) hit the ground and absorb the impact, respectively.

Of the 3, it is heel-striking that puts you at most risk of running related injuries especially if you're overweight. This is because the entire force of the impact of your body landing on the ground is absorbed by your knee joints. This is what often causes a running injury or condition known as the "runner's knee."

If you want to get a clearer picture of what I'm talking about, I want you to stop reading this book for a moment and try to jump twice. On the first jump, do so as high as you can and notice how you naturally landed on your feet. On the second attempt, jump for about an inch or two above the ground only but this time, make a conscious effort to land on your heels instead. Go ahead, drop this book and perform the 2 jumps as instructed.

I want you to take note of how each jump felt on both your ankles and your knees. Which jump felt more force or impact on the knees and ankles? That's right - the 2nd jump. And this despite jumping only 1 to 2 inches above ground! Without going into too much technical mumbo jumbo, that's the reason why you should avoid heel-striking when you run: to minimize impact on the knees and ankles. When you're able to do that, you minimize your risks of injuries and will be able to extend your running career until most people have already passed away due to old age - just like Harriette did!

Now that you know how not to hit the ground when you run, it's time to learn how to actually do it! The best way or ways to do so would be mid and/or forefoot-striking. Personally though, I prefer forefoot striking as it minimizes the impact on the knees and ankles. With mid-foot striking, you can still remove a big chunk of the impact on your knees and ankles compared to mid-foot striking with the added benefit of less strain on your calf muscles. So, I'd say alternating between the two - especially during much longer runs - may be your best bet. But if you choose to stick to just one for simplicity's sake, you'll still be able to substantially reduce risks of running injuries and extend your running longevity.

How can you learn to make forefoot or mid-foot running a natural habit? First, I want you to take off your shoes or slippers now and run across the room as if you're chasing a toddler around. Go ahead - do it now!

What did you notice? Wasn't it natural for you to run "on your toes" and employ a forefoot striking running technique? This is what the book "Born to Run" pointed out in one of its chapters that we are born to run safely and naturally using a forefoot striking technique. It's as if your feet have a mind of their own. So, when you start running later in the day or tomorrow, always remember how it felt to run barefoot across the room. That's how you should strike your feet when you run, even when you're wearing running shoes.

How about the mid-foot strike? The best way I can teach you how to employ the technique is to pay attention to where your feet land when you run. Put on your running shoes, go out and run for about 50 meters at normal pace and observe where your feet land with every stride. Drop this book now, wear your shoes, and run outside for 50 meters. Do it now!

If your lead foot lands in front of your body with each stride, you are no doubt heel striking. If that's the case, run again, but this time, make a conscious effort to land your lead foot directly beneath your body. Go ahead, do it now!

Did you notice that as your foot landed just beneath your body that the impact or the force seems much less compared to when your lead foot landed in front of you? Did you notice too that it was much easier on your ankles and knees? And that, my friend, is how you employ the mid-foot striking technique.

For proper form, you can use either forefoot or mid-foot. You can even use them both on an alternating basis. Just avoid using the heel-strike method, especially if you're overweight.

Distance and Duration

There's no fixed rule as to how long you should run as you begin training as it's dependent on your current fitness level. What you'll need to do first is to establish your baseline or starting level. To do this, go for a run for the next 3 days. Run only at a pace or speed that's comfortable for you and record both the length of time you're able to sustain your run without having to walk and the distance. For distance, you'll need to use a GPS-capable running app such as Runkeeper or Strava. Get your average time and distance and you'll get a fairly good estimate of your baseline level on which you can evaluate your training progress.

Before you run and estimate your baseline distance and duration, I want to remind you that you must learn proper running form first. When it comes to training for running long distances, your priorities should be form, distance/duration and speed, in that particular order of importance.

To increase distance and duration gradually, one of the best ways to do that is to employ the run-walk method, which was conceptualized by renowned running guru Jeff Galloway. The run-walk method is a running method whereby you run for a pre-determined number of minutes before slowing down to walk for another pre-determined number of minutes, which is usually 1 minute. Most running newbies who have no previous exercise experience whatsoever start with 1:1 running cycle, i.e., 1 minute of running followed by 1 minute of walking. As the 1:1 cycle starts to become comfortable or easy, it can be increased to 2:1, 3:1, then finally 4:1, which is the maximum cycle recommended under the technique.

The logic behind this running technique is by giving your legs a mandatory break from running, even if you're not yet dead tired, you give them the opportunity to recover faster and extend your total running distance and time. If you wait until your legs are dead tired before you give them a break, it may be too late to recover significantly and as a result, you won't be able to run as long both in terms of time and distance. In fact, many seasoned running veterans registered new personal records (PR) in terms of their running times - they were able to finish their marathons faster - when they incorporated the run-walk method. If not new PRs, many were able to finish their races feeling less tired and sore.

Start with a 1:1 cycle and increase up to 4:1 as soon as your body starts becoming accustomed to or comfortable with the current run-walk cycle. And simultaneous with this, you must also increase your current running mileage by at least 30% every month to make substantial progress and eventually finish your first 5-kilometer race in no time at all.

Speed

Your running speed has 2 components: cadence and stride. Cadence refers to how many steps or strides you take per minute. When talking about stride, we're referring to the length of your stride. Let's talk about cadence first.

When it comes to cadence and risks for running related injuries, the higher (more steps or strides per minute) the better. When your cadence is higher, your feet spend less time on the ground and that means the amount of time they have to bear the impact of the weight of your body is also much shorter. The less time the impact of your bodyweight is on your feet, the less stressed they become physically and the lower the risks of long-term injuries are. Consequently, a very slow cadence means your feet have to bear the impact of your bodyweight for much longer periods, which increases your risks of injuries over the long term.

Many running experts agree that the ideal cadence is around 170 strides or steps per minute. If you find it too fast at the start, don't worry. You can gradually build up your cadence as your training progresses. The important thing is you continuously progress towards the 170 strides per minute cadence speed. And the faster your cadence is, the faster your average running pace becomes.

As with distance and duration, it's important to get a baseline reading of your starting cadence. To do this, run for 30 seconds at your normal pace and cadence and count the number of strides or steps you take during those 30 seconds. Multiply the number by 2 and you'll get a baseline measure of your cadence.

To gradually build up your cadence towards 170 per minute, download cadence apps such as Audiostep, BeatRun, Metronome and Cadence Timer. Apps like these play a metronome that you can set and play while you run. You can time your strides to coincide with each beat that the metronome app sounds so you don't have to think about calculating your current cadence. If your baseline cadence is 130 strides per minute, you can set your cadence app's metronome speed to 135 and time your strides along with it. Once you've become comfortable with the 135 cadence after several runs, increase it to 140, and so on until you eventually reach 170 strides per minute.

The second component of running speed is the stride itself. As mentioned earlier in the section on proper form, your lead foot must always land beneath your body, regardless of whether you employ a forefoot or a mid-foot strike. In this case, how can you make your stride longer without overextending your foot in front of your body and heel strike?

You can lean your body a bit more forward, which will force you to take bigger strides but still land your lead foot at your body's center of gravity. This will make you naturally strike the ground with your mid-foot or forefoot. Work on increasing your stride only after you've achieved the 170 strides-per-minute cadence because cadence is the more crucial component for running faster.

Shoes

This is a topic that many runners are divided on. There are debates on whether or not to use stability, neutral or motion control, all of which tend to address a runner's foot pronation or the way the feet are angled as it hits the ground. Then there's the debate on whether or not minimalist (thinly or barely cushioned) shoes are much better for running longevity than maximalist (thickly cushioned) shoes.

If you use proper running form, i.e., a mid-foot or a forefoot strike, pronation won't be an issue. Why? Because your foot pronation is largely a function of how you stand or land on your heels. But if you employ a mid-foot or forefoot running technique, you take away the heel strike and thus, pronation wouldn't even be an issue.

How can I say that? When I first started running, I didn't know that mid-foot and forefoot strikes even existed. All I knew was to land on my heels and roll my foot with each stride. And as I became more enamored with running, I started to read about pronation and types of running shoes for pronation. I had my gait analyzed at a top-end running store and found that I needed to use a stability type of running shoe given my feet's pronation. So, I got a stability running shoe and continued heel strike running.

As my running distance increased over the next year or so, I started to feel some discomfort in my knees. I figured it was because I was overweight. Then I chanced upon a book that would forever change the way I ran - Christopher McDougall's best-selling book "Born to Run." Through that book, I learned about another way of running - the forefoot striking technique. In that book as well, I learned about how useful minimalist running shoes can be for forefoot running - how it actually makes it easier and more natural to use a forefoot striking technique with minimalist running shoes versus running in a thickly-cushioned (maximalist) pair of running shoes. And by its minimalist nature, minimalist running shoes only come in one variety - the neutral type that offers no pronation support whatsoever.

Despite being a "stability shoe person," I ran exclusively in minimalist running shoes for the next several years because of what I learned through the book. In particular, I used the Nike

Free line of running shoes. Lo and behold, the knee discomfort disappeared and I actually started to run faster. Plus, I developed my calf muscles really well! Then I registered to run my first marathon.

As I was training for my first marathon, my running coach recommended I try a pair of Hoka One One Clifton 3 running shoes. Hoka is a Maori (New Zealand) brand of specialized running shoes that re-ignited the maximalist shoe craze after it died down due to the minimalist trend. So, I went to a specialty running store to check it out.

But before asking for the Hokas, I asked to have my gait analyzed first as I already forgot if I was a "stability" or "motion control" runner. To my surprise, my gait changed to "neutral" after all those years of running in minimalist shoes. Then I went to check out the Hokas.

Seeing how thick the soles were, I already discounted using them for my runs because from what I understood, most thick-soled and well-cushioned running shoes tend to promote a heel strike technique. But curiosity got the better of me and I tried it on the treadmill of the running store I visited.

Whoa - I never imagined running in a well-cushioned maximalist shoe could actually promote a mid-foot/forefoot striking technique! In fact, it was quite uncomfortable to heel strike using the Hoka Clifton 3s, making it natural for me to employ a mid-foot or forefoot technique - with lots of cushioning to boot! It helped me run much longer almost immediately because of the added cushioning comfort without sacrificing proper running form.

It doesn't really matter if you use minimalist or maximalist shoes. What I discovered to be the key to naturally gravitate towards a mid-foot or forefoot strike is the difference between the thickness of the running shoe's soles at the toe area and the heel area, which referred to as the heel-to-toe drop. At most, the clearance between the ground-toes and the ground-heel areas is zero, meaning they're equal.

The problem with most thickly-cushioned running shoes is that most of the cushioning lies in the heel area, making its clearance from the ground much higher than that of the toe area, i.e., the sole is sloped downward from heel to the toe hence the term heel-to-toe drop. That makes it very easy and natural to heel-strike and very hard, if not impossible, to employ a mid-foot or a forefoot strike. The Hokas I used - that pair of maximalist shoes - had a very small or practically non-existent heel-to-toe drop, which made it feel natural to run with a mid-foot or forefoot striking technique. And it's the same reason why minimalist shoes promote the same techniques - a low heel-to-toe drop.

Complementary Training

When it comes to increasing your running stamina and speed, you'll need to develop muscular endurance and cardiovascular fitness. Another way to increase both without over training is to incorporate other cardio exercises in between your running training. Two of the best complementary exercises for your running training program are biking and swimming. We'll take a look at how to best incorporate them later on at the end of Chapter 6.

Chapter 4 - Rest

The second important aspect of being able to effectively achieve your 5K minimum running distance and become fitter in the process is getting enough rest. While it may seem to be common sense to get enough rest, this is one topic that many people don't really understand or appreciate. Hence in this chapter, we'll discuss about how rest plays a very important role in your fitness goals and what it really means to get enough of it.

Why Rest?

One of the best reasons for getting enough rest is you can recharge your mind. More than just physical power, you'll need all the mental (specifically, willpower) strength you can muster to break the inertia of a sedentary lifestyle and start training regularly to be able to run at least 5K and become a fit person, especially on those very cold mornings when waking up early to go for a run is akin to lifting a 1,000-pound barbell. When you get enough rest, you give your mind the chance to replenish its willpower reserves, which is a limited resource, contrary to popular opinion.

When you get enough rest on a regular basis, you can actually do more during your training sessions, i.e., work out much harder. Believe it or not, the quality of your training is directly affected by the quality of your recovery, which getting enough rest. If you give your body enough time off from physical training to just recover, you allow it to become stronger and train harder and better.

And more than just being able to train harder, you'll be able to train more and more consistently. One of the reasons many people fail to follow through on their running training programs is because, at some point, they felt too tired to continue, i.e., burned out. When you give both your body and mind adequate and regular rest in between workouts, you minimize the chances of not being able to work out again the next time, which in turn increases your chances of being able to train consistently. And its consistently smaller gains that will allow you to successfully achieve your running goals, not one-time-big-time Herculean workouts.

Getting enough rest also allows you to minimize your risks for getting injured. In particular, you reduce your body's risks for overtraining-related injuries like stress fractures and tendonitis. And when you're perfectly healthy - i.e., injury-free - and are able to train consistently at a high level, you'll be able to run longer and faster, which will ultimately make you a very fit person!

And speaking of getting fit, many people make the mistake of believing that fitness or fitness gains are achieved during training. The truth is much of your running-related training gains will come as a direct result of getting enough rest in between trainings. Your body will need enough time to adapt to the stress that you put it through during trainings and such adaptations occur during periods of rest, not activity. Activity triggers your body to adapt and the actual adaptation occurs during rest.

How to Get Enough Rest and Recovery

The very first thing you'll need to do is get enough sleep. Being chronically sleep-deficient is one of the best ways to sabotage not just your running training but just about any worthwhile endeavor you're into. More than just physical, lack of sleep can also weaken you mentally - deplete your willpower and make it easier for you to ditch training frequently or worse, quit altogether.

So how much sleep do you really need? Some people swear by getting only 4 hours of sleep every night while some say they need an average of 10 hours nightly! And that's on top of what many "experts" say - that 8 hours on average should be your goal.

I'd say that 8 hours may be a good place to start but the best way to estimate your sleeping hour requirements is by how you generally feel on most days. Here's what I suggest you do for the next 7 days that can help you get a very good estimate of your sleeping requirements.

Every night before going to bed, write down what time you hit the sack. When you wake up in the morning, write down what time you woke up, how many hours of sleep you got, how you felt when you woke up and how well you slept that night. And at the end of the day, preferably before hitting the sack again, write down how you generally felt throughout the day, e.g., sleepy, energetic, sluggish, unable to focus, laser-like focus and determination, etc.

After 7 days, read through what you wrote. Take note of the days when you felt generally energetic and focused throughout the day, what time you slept the night before, what time you woke up and how you felt throughout the day. From there, you can get a pretty good estimate of how many hours of sleep you need and what time in the evening and morning you should hit the sack and wake up, respectively.

Another thing you'll need to consider about rest is physical rest, i.e., the amount of time your leg muscles need to rest before running again. A good general guideline is to give your muscles about 48 hours of rest before working them out again. This means if you ran today, you should run again 2 days from now. That can give your leg muscles enough time to recover from the previous workout's challenges and stresses, which can optimize the speed at which you progress in your running training.

Possible Signs That You're Not Getting Enough Rest

When you start training for your first 5K and beyond, it'll be very hard - if not impossible - to detect if you're overtraining already and aren't able to get enough rest until it's too late. But if you know the red flags, you can catch it early on and make the necessary adjustments so you can get enough rest to avoid getting burned out or over trained.

The following are red flags you'll need to watch out for that may indicate overtraining and lack of rest:
- Extra tightness or soreness in your leg muscles that persists for several days;
- You feel tired for extended periods of time after several training sessions;

- You're not able to give as much effort (speed or duration) compared to previous workouts despite feeling that you've been putting in more effort;
- You're voraciously craving for much more food than usual, especially processed and high sugar foods just to give you a fast energy boost;
- Your motivation to train has been dipping significantly and your patience seems to be very thin lately; and
- Your resting heart rate in the morning is higher by an average of 5 to 10 heartbeats.

What can you do to reverse your low energy levels? If necessary, take an occasional extra day or two off from training. The key word here is occasional and for optimal results, it's best to stick to three times per week training.

If you don't want to break your momentum, you can instead cut back on your training volume or intensity. Instead of completing 10 cycles per your schedule for example, cut back to 6 to 8 cycles instead, depending on how tired you feel. That way, you strike a comfortable middle ground wherein you don't break your momentum but don't continue overtraining your body.

Another way to avoid breaking momentum without continuing to over train is to substitute one of your running workouts with a complementary cardio workout, i.e., biking or swimming at a comfortable pace for 20 to 30 minutes. They don't work the legs out as much as running but it still trains your cardiovascular system, which is a crucial component for running too.

One possible reason for being low in energy despite getting enough sleep and at least 48 hours of recovery is poor post-training nutrition. We'll discuss this more in Chapter 5 but suffice to say, you will need to get enough calories immediately after your training to kick start the recovery process as soon as possible.

Lastly, you can add more hours to your sleep for 1 or 2 nights straight. Especially in the beginning, the body needs more time to recover during sleep as it starts to acclimatize itself to the new stresses placed upon it as a result of regular running. As your body adapts to the new stress and routine, your normal sleeping hours will return.

Chapter 5 - Nutrition

To excel in any sport, you will need to watch your diet. Whether it's running, bodybuilding or playing football, your diet will determine to a large extent whether or not you can perform optimally for sustained periods of time. While a very nutritious diet that is chock full of nutrients won't necessarily make you as fast as Usain Bolt, a very good diet or nutrition plan can significantly improve your health and your immune system, which can allow you to train harder for longer periods of time.

When it comes to calories, there are three general types, also referred to as macronutrients. These are carbohydrates, protein and fat. More than just providing your body with the necessary amount of energy for running, you need the necessary nutrition for basic physiological processes that can significantly impact your ability to train and to run.

When it comes to optimal running nutrition, a balanced and healthy diet is needed. What this means is your diet should be able to provide most if not all of your nutrient needs, which can lead to excellent health and improved performance. Speaking of nutrients, be wary of claims that a specific vitamin or nutrient taken in very large servings will lead to supernatural performance results. That's hogwash - overall health and performance are only achieved via a holistic and healthy diet together with optimal training.

What You Need To Eat

When talking about optimal nutrition, the main topic is always what to eat. By simply focusing on what to eat for optimal performance and health, you already eliminate foods that you shouldn't be eating. In contrast, focusing on what not to eat will still require you to think about what is best to eat. And for the top food items when it comes to training for your first 5K run and becoming fit, here are some of the food items you'll need to focus on more:

Complex Carbohydrates

In just about any sport, getting enough of the right kind of carbohydrates is crucial for optimal performance. Why? It's because complex carbohydrates take time to break down in the stomach and, as such, enter the bloodstream in a more steady and consistent pace. As such, complex carbohydrates provide sustained energy without subsequent crashes, like what normally happens when you load up on simple carbohydrates (e.g., sugary foods and other "white" carbs). The best sources of complex carbohydrates for training for your first 5K include unrefined pastas, sweet potatoes, veggies, whole wheat breads, and brown rice. Anything else, keep to small, infrequent amounts throughout the week, i.e., occasional treats or rewards.

You can consume high sugar foods, (when I say this I mean natural sugars such as what you find in most fruits) only within the first 15 minutes after you ended your run or training. Why is this? It's because this is the most opportune time when your muscles are in need of fast acting carbohydrates. In particular, it's during this window that your muscles can immediately replenish their spent-up glycogen stores.

Your carbohydrate intake must comprise about 60% of your diet as a runner. This is because of the huge energy demand from running training.

Protein

When you train your leg muscles the way you do when running, you create micro tears in your legs' muscles' fibers, which is a normal part of any physical training. The longer your runs become, the more muscle fibers can be "torn" and will require adequate repair en route to running performance improvements.

When it comes to muscle repair and growth, nothing else is as important as protein. This is your muscle cell's basic building blocks. A good guideline for how much protein you'll need as you train for running your first 5K and beyond is to consume at least 1.5 grams of protein per kilogram of bodyweight. So, if you weigh 100 kilos, you'll need 150 grams of protein daily. If you weigh only 50 kilos, then you'll need to consume 75 grams of protein every day.

Some of the best sources of lean protein, which is important if you're overweight, are skinless chicken breasts, egg whites, fish, and lean cuts of beef. Always look for how the animals were fed, for the most part if possible buy organic products. Proteins should comprise no more than 20% of your daily caloric consumption.

Dietary Fats

Not all dietary fats are created equal so for consuming this macronutrient, you must choose wisely. More so that of all the 3 macronutrients, the 2 others being carbs and protein, dietary fat is the most calorie-dense at 9 calories per gram vs. only 4 calories per gram for both carbs and protein.

When it comes to dietary fat, what you should focus on are monounsaturated fats, also referred to as healthy fats. This type of dietary fat is what makes both the Okinawa and Mediterranean diets very effective in lowering risks of cardiovascular diseases despite their very high fat content. So, as a runner, it's best for you to get your daily fat fix from flax seed oil, canola oil, olive oil and avocados instead of lard or fast foods that are deep fried. Dietary fat calories shouldn't exceed 20% of your daily total consumption.

Vitamins and Minerals

Next to getting enough of the Big Three (macronutrients), vitamins and minerals are the next most important members of your nutrition team. You can think of them as bench or role players if you will, which can prove to be very crucial for successfully building up your endurance, performance and, consequently, your fitness.

Because you'll be exercising or training regularly for your first 5K race, your daily caloric requirements will definitely need to increase - and that will entail more vitamins and minerals too. And while vitamins and minerals in supplement form will never really make up for a diet that's very poor in vitamins and minerals like Vitamins C, A, E and Zinc, they will also play a huge role in your ability to get enough vitamins and minerals because these days, it can be very hard to get everything from whole foods. The key here is to always remember that as supplements, that's what they really are - just "extras" or additions to what is already a healthy and nutrition-filled diet.

Hydration

If the ordinary, average person who doesn't exercise needs to get enough water on a daily basis, can you imagine how much more important it is for people who exercise on a regular basis? And when it comes to being properly hydrated, you must aim to drink up to 8 cups daily - or about 2 liters a day. And while caffeinated drinks like teas, coffee and - God forbid - energy drinks and alcohol may be counted as fluids for hydration's sake, it's important to keep in mind that caffeine is a natural diuretic, i.e., it flushes fluids out of your body. As such, it's best to minimize them or limit their consumption while increasing fluid intake.

So how do you know if you're well hydrated? Your urine is a very good indicator. If it's clear to light yellow in color, you're adequately hydrated. If it's dark yellow, you're dehydrated.

Meal Replacements

In today's very busy world, eating healthy meals can be quite challenging. For those moments where getting in enough quality calories for a run can be very challenging or impossible to do with whole foods, you can go for meal replacement shakes. Especially before going for a run, it can even be a much better alternative to eating real food because it's much easier on your stomach for digestion. A good meal replacement should also include whey protein and not just carbs.

On Snacking

One of the things that you will definitely notice as you continue in your training for your first 5K run is your metabolism. In particular, you'll find that it will become faster, i.e., your body will start burning more and more calories as you progress in your training program. And this means you'll get hungrier more often.

The best way to deal with hunger pangs isn't to use willpower to resist it but to satisfy it with a healthy alternative - healthy snacking! Some of the best snacks to munch on in between your meals include protein bars, eggs, nuts, fruit and veggie smoothies, whole grain sandwiches made from lean turkey or chicken breast, and fresh fruit and veggies. By eating healthy in between meals, you can ensure that your body gets enough quality calories to power you through your 5K run training. Avoid processed and sugary treats like donuts, bagels, cereals and the like for snacks. Most of its sugar and empty calories.

Plan all Eating

It's been said that failing to plan is planning for failure. When you don't eat enough, you won't have enough energy and nutrients for training consistently and effectively. If you eat too much, it can be just as detrimental to your training.

So, what are the things you'll need to plan for when it comes to optimum nutrition for running? One is to make sure that you'll be able to feed your body enough quality calories on a daily basis. Especially if you live a very busy lifestyle or have to work or go to school every day, you will need to have a plan to make sure such kinds of food are readily available to you all throughout the day. And this may mean you'll have to identify nearby restaurants or establishments that offer healthy whole foods. And if there are none, you may have to plan on preparing food at home that you can take along with you that you can conveniently eat wherever you go.

Another thing you'll need to plan well ahead for is the timing of your meals. In particular, you'll need to eat a meal that's loaded with complex carbs 3 hours prior to your planned run, as this will ensure you'll have energy to complete it without abdominal discomfort.   The best pre-run complex carb sources are oatmeal, bananas, porridge, whole-wheat bread, brown rice and sweet potatoes.

And for your post run meals, you must consume simple carbs (a valid reason to eat relatively sugary foods) together with fast acting protein (whey protein is best) within the first 2 hours after your run (the so-called Golden Window) to aid in recovery and muscle repair.

Chapter 6 - Your 12-Week Plan To Finish Your First 5K

Okay, here's where the rubber meets the road. We've extensively covered your 12-week running program's important principles, the basic but important foundations on which you must build your running endurance, distance and eventually speed. Now, I'll be laying the smack down on what'll be your 12-week running plan for finishing your first 5-kilometer run.

But before I do that, I want you to know the 3 most important things you must go for during these 12 weeks:
- You must train consistently at least 3 times weekly;
- You must always prioritize in this order - proper running form, distance, and speed; and
- You should never train with an injury or pain.

That being said, let's get down to it! Oh wait, I forgot one more thing: This running plan is meant for total newbies so it will not be as "challenging" in the first week or two. However, since you'll be starting at your estimated running base (Chapter 3 on Distance), the running plan can still work well for you if you've already got some running experience behind you. Just adjust your running distances accordingly.

Week 1

The first week is crucial for you, especially if you're a total newbie. Why? If you train too hard or too long, you may abhor the whole running thing altogether pand just quit. But if it's too easy, you may not progress as much. That's why you'll need to train at just the right level by starting at your estimated baseline level that you learned to measure in Chapter 3.

Before we do this, it's important that you use a GPS-enabled running app like Runkeeper or Strava so you can have an objective basis to evaluate your progress or lack thereof. Evaluating your running progress by basing it simply on how you feel is a very poor way of doing so as feelings ebb and tide, which make for unstable and subjective assessments of progress.

As mentioned earlier, you will need to train 3 times weekly and should have about 48 hours rest for your leg muscles in between workouts for optimal recovery. Many people choose an M-W-F or T-Th-S schedule.

For the actual training itself, you will do the Run-Walk method discussed earlier in Chapter 3 and, in particular, you can start with the 1:1 protocol, i.e., run at your comfortable pace for 1 minute, walk for 1 minute, and repeat the cycle 10 times for a total workout time of 20 minutes. Remember to warm up first by walking around the block for 5 minutes and doing dynamic stretches for another 5, which was explained in Chapter 3.

Week 2

Now that you've broken yourself into the world of running with the 1:1 Run-Walk protocol, it's time to increase your duration/distance by adding 2 more cycles from 10 to 12, which will increase total workout time to 24 minutes. Warm up properly and cool down before and after working out, respectively.

Week 3

For this week, it's time to add one more minute to the running part, i.e., you'll now use the 2:1 Run-Walk protocol, i.e., run or jog for 2 minutes at your comfortable pace and walk for 1 minute, and repeat 8 times. The decrease in number of cycles from 12 to 8 will be compensated for by the increase in your running duration from 1 minute to 2 minutes per cycle. While the total workout time will remain at 24 minutes, your effective workout time will go up to 16 minutes from only 12 minutes the week prior.

Remember to warm up and cool down properly at the end of every workout.

Week 4

For this week's workout, you'll maintain the current 2:1 running protocol but increase total cycles from 8 to 10, which will increase total and effective workout times to 30 minutes and 20 minutes, respectively per workout. Don't forget to warm up and cool down properly.

Week 5

For your workouts during the week, increase the running portion to 3 minutes, shifting to a 3:1 Run-Walk protocol, reducing the cycle to just 8. However, this will increase your total workout duration by 2 minutes to 32 minutes per workout and increase your effective workout time to 24 minutes from only 20 the week before. Remember to warm up and cool down before and after your workouts, respectively.

Week 6

For the 6th week, maintain the 3:1 protocol but increase the cycles to 10, which will increase both total and effective workout times to 40 minutes and 30 minutes, respectively. Don't forget to warm up and cool down properly. At this point, you should be able to complete between 3.8 to 4.3 kilometers in 40 minutes of Run-Walking.

Week 7

For this week, increase the running protocol to 4:1, i.e., 4 minutes run and 1 minute walk and perform 8 cycles only. While total workout time remains at 40 minutes, your effective workout time will increase to 32 minutes and so will your running distance. As always, warm up and cool down properly.

Week 8

Given that you've already achieved the maximum recommended protocol of 4:1, it's time to up the ante on your duration and by consequence, distance. Increase your Run-Walk cycles from 8 cycles to at least 9, for a total workout time of 45 minutes and effective workout time of 36 minutes. At this point, you'd be running anywhere from 4 to 4.5 kilometers already.

And it's even possible - depending on the rate at which your running speed has been progressing - that you're already completing a 5-kilometer run by now. If so, the remaining 4 weeks will allow you to exceed the 5-kilometer minimum goal!

Again, warm up and cool down properly.

Weeks 9 to 12

Increase your Run-Walk cycles to at least 10, increasing your total and effective workout times to 50 minutes. At this point, you'd have completed 5 kilometers already and you just add 1 or 2 cycles more if by the end of your 50-minute workouts, you're running app still registers a sub-5-kilometer total distance. And once you've already reached or exceeded your 5-kilometer goal, you can decide whether or not to stick to current cycle number, reduce it (particularly if you want to maintain the 5-kilometer distance but run at a faster speed), or increase it (to add gradually add to your running mileage).

For Running the Distance

If you've already started to finish 5 to 10 kilometers on a regular basis and would like to up the ante and go for a half marathon (21 kilometers) or even a full marathon (42 kilometers), you can incorporate complimentary exercises in between your workouts. In particular, you can incorporate swimming and/or biking.

If your running schedule is M-W-F, you can incorporate swimming on Tuesday, Thursday, Saturday or Sunday. While if you plan to bike, you can best incorporate it on Sunday then adjust your training schedule for next week to T-Th-S. Why?

Because compared to swimming, biking primarily works out your leg muscles. And given the 48-hour minimum recovery guideline, your next running workout must be on Tuesday.

How long should you perform these complementary workouts? 30 to 40 minutes is a good place to start. Adjust the duration accordingly if needed.

Conclusion

Thank you for buying this book! I hope that through it you've learned so much about how to achieve your fitness goals via running. But more importantly I hope that it has encouraged you to take action by applying what you learned here and start lacing up your running shoes and hitting the road to start training for your first 5K run. You see, knowing is just half the battle and for a complete victory, knowledge needs to be applied. With the 12-week beginner's 5K running plan I've outlined for you, I've taken the burden of guesswork from you so you can just focus on executing the running plan.

Here's to your running success my friend! Cheers!

Website References:

1. http://womensrunning.competitor.com/2017/10/news/harriette-thompson-oldest-woman-run-marathon-half-passes-away-94_81779

2. https://www.runnersworld.com/older-runners/harriette-thompson-oldest-woman-to-finish-a-marathon-dies-at-94

3. https://therunningbug.com/fitness/tips-and-advice/the-importance-of-rest-and-recovery

4. https://www.realbuzz.com/articles-interests/running/article/7-reasons-why-rest-and-recovery-are-important/

5. https://www.active.com/running/articles/nutrition-tips-for-new-runners

6. https://www.active.com/running/articles/nutrition-tips-for-new-runners?page=2